Precision Engineering: Exploring Genetic Engineering and Gene Therapy Techniques for Engineers

Dawson Knox

Copyright © [2023]

Title: Precision Engineering: Exploring Genetic Engineering and Gene Therapy Techniques for Engineers

Author's: Dawson Knox

All rights reserved. No part of this publication may be reproduced, stored in a retrieval system, or transmitted in any form or by any means, electronic, mechanical, photocopying, recording, or otherwise, without the prior written permission of the publisher or author, except in the case of brief quotations embodied in critical reviews and certain other non-commercial uses permitted by copyright law.

This book was printed and published by [Publisher's: **Dawson Knox**] in [2023]

ISBN:

TABLE OF CONTENT

Chapter 1: Introduction to Genetic Engineering and Gene Therapy 07

Overview of Genetic Engineering

Historical Background

Importance of Genetic Engineering in Engineering Field

Chapter 2: Fundamentals of Genetics and Molecular Biology 14

Basics of Genetics

DNA Structure and Replication

Gene Expression and Regulation

Chapter 3: Tools and Techniques in Genetic Engineering 21

Recombinant DNA Technology

Polymerase Chain Reaction (PCR)

DNA Sequencing and Analysis

Gene Cloning and Expression

Chapter 4: Genetic Engineering Applications in Engineering 30

Genetic Modification of Microorganisms

Genetic Engineering in Agriculture

Industrial Applications

Environmental Applications

Chapter 5: Introduction to Gene Therapy 39

Understanding Gene Therapy

Types of Gene Therapy

Challenges and Ethical Considerations in Gene Therapy

Chapter 6: Gene Delivery Systems 45

Viral Vectors

Non-viral Vectors

Advancements in Gene Delivery Systems

Chapter 7: Gene Editing Techniques　　52

CRISPR-Cas9 System

Zinc Finger Nucleases (ZFNs)

Transcription Activator-Like Effector Nucleases (TALENs)

Chapter 8: Applications of Gene Therapy in Engineering　　58

Gene Therapy for Genetic Disorders

Gene Therapy for Cancer

Gene Therapy in Tissue Engineering

Future Possibilities and Innovations in Gene Therapy

Chapter 9: Regulatory and Safety Considerations in Genetic Engineering and Gene Therapy　　66

Ethical Guidelines for Genetic Engineering

Regulatory Bodies and Approval Processes

Safety Measures and Risk Assessment

Chapter 10: Case Studies and Success Stories in Genetic Engineering and Gene Therapy   74

Case Study 1: Successful Gene Therapy Treatment

Case Study 2: Genetic Engineering Breakthrough in Engineering Field

Case Study 3: Gene Editing in Biomedical Engineering

Chapter 11: Future Perspectives and Emerging Technologies in Genetic Engineering   81

Advancements in Gene Editing Techniques

Synthetic Biology and Genetic Engineering

Nanotechnology in Genetic Engineering

Chapter 12: Conclusion and Final Thoughts   88

Recapitulation of Key Concepts

Importance of Genetic Engineering and Gene Therapy for Engineers

Future Potential and Challenges in the Field

Chapter 1: Introduction to Genetic Engineering and Gene Therapy

Overview of Genetic Engineering

Genetic engineering is a revolutionary field in biomedical science and biotechnology that has the potential to transform the way we approach healthcare and disease prevention. This subchapter provides engineers with an overview of the principles, techniques, and applications of genetic engineering, highlighting its significance in advancing precision engineering.

At its core, genetic engineering involves the manipulation and modification of an organism's genetic material, specifically its DNA. Through precise and controlled methods, scientists are able to introduce new genes, alter existing ones, or remove unwanted genes altogether. This capability allows for the creation of organisms with desired traits or the correction of genetic defects that cause diseases.

One of the fundamental techniques used in genetic engineering is recombinant DNA technology. This involves the extraction and isolation of specific genes from one organism and their insertion into another organism, resulting in the production of recombinant DNA. This process has paved the way for a wide range of applications, including the development of genetically modified organisms (GMOs), production of therapeutic proteins, and gene therapy.

Engineers play a vital role in the field of genetic engineering by designing and optimizing the tools and techniques used in the laboratory. They contribute to developing innovative technologies such as DNA sequencing, gene editing, and gene delivery systems. Precision engineering principles are essential in ensuring the accuracy, efficiency, and safety of these techniques.

Genetic engineering has already made significant contributions to various areas of biomedicine. For instance, the production of therapeutic proteins, such as insulin, in bacterial or mammalian cells has revolutionized the treatment of diabetes. Additionally, gene therapy approaches are being explored to address genetic disorders by replacing or repairing defective genes.

Furthermore, genetic engineering is instrumental in the development of genetically modified crops that are resistant to pests, diseases, or environmental stressors. This has the potential to enhance food production and reduce the reliance on harmful pesticides and herbicides.

However, the field of genetic engineering also raises various ethical, legal, and social concerns. Engineers need to be aware of these issues and ensure responsible and ethical practices in their work. This includes considerations such as the potential risks associated with genetically modified organisms, privacy concerns with genetic data, and fair access to genetic technologies.

In conclusion, genetic engineering is a powerful tool that holds immense potential for advancements in biomedicine and biotechnology. Engineers play a critical role in driving this field forward by developing precise and efficient techniques. Understanding the principles and applications of genetic engineering is essential for engineers in the biomedical science and biotechnology niches, as it provides the foundation for innovative solutions to complex healthcare challenges.

Historical Background

In the world of precision engineering, the field of genetic engineering and gene therapy stands out as a revolutionary force in the realms of biomedical science and biotechnology. To fully appreciate the advancements and breakthroughs achieved in this field, it is crucial to delve into its historical background.

The origins of genetic engineering can be traced back to the early 1970s when the scientific community witnessed a groundbreaking discovery. In 1973, scientists Stanley Cohen and Herbert Boyer successfully isolated a gene from one organism and inserted it into another, marking the birth of recombinant DNA technology. This pivotal moment paved the way for manipulating and altering genetic material, thereby opening up endless possibilities in the field of genetic engineering.

Rapid progress continued in the late 1970s, with the development of techniques such as restriction enzymes, DNA sequencing, and polymerase chain reaction (PCR). These breakthroughs allowed scientists to manipulate DNA with greater precision and accuracy, enabling the creation of genetically modified organisms (GMOs) and the study of gene function.

The 1980s saw the birth of gene therapy, a branch of genetic engineering aimed at treating genetic disorders by introducing functional genes into patients' cells. The first successful gene therapy trial occurred in 1990, where a four-year-old girl with severe immune deficiency was treated using genetically modified cells. While the field faced setbacks and ethical dilemmas in the following years, it laid the groundwork for further advancements in gene therapy.

The Human Genome Project, initiated in 1990, was a monumental endeavor that aimed to map and sequence the entire human genome. Completed in 2003, this project provided scientists with a comprehensive understanding of the genetic makeup of humans, leading to significant breakthroughs in personalized medicine and the identification of disease-causing genes.

Today, precision engineering techniques in genetic engineering and gene therapy have advanced by leaps and bounds. The advent of CRISPR-Cas9 technology in the early 2010s revolutionized the field, allowing scientists to precisely edit genes with unprecedented ease, speed, and accuracy. This powerful tool has opened doors to potential treatments for previously incurable diseases, such as cancer, HIV, and genetic disorders.

As engineers in the fields of biomedical science and biotechnology, it is essential to comprehend the historical context of precision engineering techniques in genetic engineering and gene therapy. Understanding the past enables us to appreciate the significance of present breakthroughs and fuels our drive to push the boundaries of what is possible in the future. By harnessing the power of precision engineering, we can continue to revolutionize the field and bring about transformative advancements in healthcare and human well-being.

Importance of Genetic Engineering in Engineering Field

Genetic engineering has emerged as a groundbreaking field with immense potential for engineering advancements, particularly in the domains of biomedical science and biotechnology. In this subchapter, we will delve into the significance of genetic engineering in the engineering field, exploring its applications, benefits, and potential challenges.

Genetic engineering, also known as genetic modification or gene manipulation, involves the alteration of an organism's genetic material to introduce new traits or enhance existing ones. This technology has revolutionized the engineering field, offering engineers unprecedented control over the genetic makeup of living organisms.

In the realm of biomedical science, genetic engineering has played a pivotal role in the development of life-saving therapies and treatments. Engineers working in this field can utilize genetic engineering techniques to create genetically modified organisms (GMOs) that produce essential pharmaceuticals, such as insulin and growth hormones. The ability to genetically engineer microorganisms has also paved the way for the production of biopharmaceuticals, including vaccines and antibodies, on a large scale.

Moreover, genetic engineering enables engineers to modify the genetic code of plants and animals, enhancing their desirable traits. This has led to the development of genetically modified crops with increased resistance to pests, diseases, and environmental stressors. These genetically modified crops not only ensure food security but also have the potential to address global challenges such as malnutrition and climate change.

In the field of biotechnology, genetic engineering has opened up new avenues for engineering applications. Engineers can now design and engineer proteins, enzymes, and other biomolecules with desired properties for use in various industrial processes. This has led to the production of biofuels, bioplastics, and other sustainable materials, reducing our reliance on fossil fuels and minimizing environmental impact.

However, while the potential of genetic engineering is immense, it also raises ethical and safety concerns. Engineers working in this field must navigate these challenges carefully, ensuring that the benefits outweigh the potential risks. Striking a balance between progress and ethical considerations is crucial to maintain public trust and ensure responsible engineering practices.

In conclusion, genetic engineering holds tremendous importance in the engineering field, particularly in the realms of biomedical science and biotechnology. The ability to manipulate genetic material provides engineers with unprecedented control and opens up new possibilities for innovation. By harnessing the power of genetic engineering, engineers can develop life-saving therapies, enhance crop productivity, and revolutionize various industrial processes. However, it is imperative to approach genetic engineering with caution, taking into account ethical and safety considerations to ensure responsible and sustainable engineering practices.

Chapter 2: Fundamentals of Genetics and Molecular Biology

Basics of Genetics

In the fast-paced world of precision engineering, it is essential for engineers to have a solid understanding of the fundamentals of genetics. This knowledge forms the foundation for exploring genetic engineering and gene therapy techniques, which have revolutionized the fields of biomedical science and biotechnology. In this subchapter, we will delve into the basics of genetics, providing engineers with a comprehensive overview of the key concepts and principles that underpin these revolutionary technologies.

Genetics is the study of genes, heredity, and the variation of traits within a population. Genes are segments of DNA that contain instructions for building and maintaining an organism. They determine our physical characteristics, such as eye color, height, and susceptibility to certain diseases. Heredity refers to the passing of genes from one generation to the next, while variation refers to the differences in traits observed among individuals.

One of the fundamental principles of genetics is the structure and function of DNA. DNA, or deoxyribonucleic acid, is a double helix molecule composed of nucleotides. These nucleotides consist of a sugar, a phosphate group, and one of four nitrogenous bases: adenine (A), thymine (T), cytosine (C), and guanine (G). The sequence of these bases forms the genetic code, which determines the unique characteristics of each individual.

Genetic traits can either be inherited through dominant or recessive genes. Dominant traits are expressed when at least one copy of the gene is present, while recessive traits require two copies of the gene for expression. Understanding the patterns of inheritance is crucial for engineers working on genetic engineering projects, as it allows them to predict the likelihood of passing on specific traits to future generations.

Furthermore, engineers must familiarize themselves with the techniques used to manipulate genes. Genetic engineering involves the alteration of an organism's genetic material to achieve desired traits or outcomes. This can be achieved through techniques such as gene cloning, gene editing, and gene transfer. These techniques have paved the way for advancements in medical treatments, agricultural practices, and environmental conservation.

By grasping the basics of genetics, engineers in the fields of biomedical science and biotechnology can effectively contribute to the development of innovative genetic engineering and gene therapy techniques. This subchapter serves as a stepping stone for engineers, providing them with the necessary knowledge to navigate the complex world of genetics and harness its potential for the betterment of society.

DNA Structure and Replication

Introduction:

In the field of precision engineering, understanding the fundamental principles of DNA structure and replication is crucial for engineers working in the biomedical science and biotechnology niches. This subchapter aims to provide a comprehensive overview of DNA structure and replication, elucidating the key concepts and mechanisms that underpin genetic engineering and gene therapy techniques. By delving into the intricacies of DNA, engineers can harness its potential to develop innovative solutions for various applications, from targeted drug delivery systems to gene editing technologies.

DNA Structure:

Deoxyribonucleic Acid (DNA) is a double-stranded helical molecule that carries the genetic information responsible for the development and functioning of all living organisms. The structure of DNA consists of two antiparallel strands, forming a double helix. Each strand comprises a linear sequence of nucleotides, which consist of a sugar-phosphate backbone and a nitrogenous base. The four nitrogenous bases include adenine (A), thymine (T), cytosine (C), and guanine (G), which pair specifically with their complementary bases (A with T and C with G). This base pairing provides the foundation for DNA replication and genetic information transfer.

DNA Replication:

DNA replication is a highly precise process that ensures the accurate transmission of genetic information from one generation to the next. It involves the duplication of the DNA molecule, allowing cells to divide and pass on their genetic material. The replication process begins with the unwinding of the DNA double helix, mediated by specialized enzymes called helicases. As the strands separate, DNA polymerases catalyze the synthesis of new complementary strands by adding nucleotides in a 5' to 3' direction. The leading strand is synthesized continuously, while the lagging strand is synthesized in short fragments called Okazaki fragments, which are later joined by DNA ligases.

Implications for Engineers:

Understanding DNA structure and replication opens up a myriad of possibilities for engineers in the biomedical science and biotechnology fields. By harnessing the knowledge of DNA, engineers can design and develop novel technologies that leverage genetic information to address various challenges. For instance, precision engineering techniques can be employed to create targeted drug delivery systems, utilizing the specific base pairing properties of DNA to guide drug molecules to desired cellular targets. Additionally, gene editing technologies, such as CRISPR-Cas9, rely on the principles of DNA structure and replication to precisely modify genetic sequences, offering immense potential for treating genetic diseases.

Conclusion:

In conclusion, DNA structure and replication form the foundation for genetic engineering and gene therapy techniques. Engineers working in the biomedical science and biotechnology niches must possess a deep understanding of these principles to drive innovation in their respective fields. By unraveling the mysteries of DNA, engineers can unlock the potential to develop cutting-edge technologies that revolutionize the diagnosis, treatment, and prevention of diseases. The knowledge gained from DNA structure and replication provides a solid framework for engineers to pioneer advancements in precision engineering, ultimately improving the quality of life for individuals worldwide.

Gene Expression and Regulation

In the world of genetic engineering and gene therapy, the understanding of gene expression and regulation plays a pivotal role. As engineers delving into the realm of biomedical science and biotechnology, it is essential to comprehend the intricate mechanisms that govern gene expression and how they can be manipulated to achieve desired outcomes.

Gene expression refers to the process by which genetic information stored in DNA is transcribed into RNA and ultimately translated into functional proteins. This process is tightly regulated at various levels to ensure that genes are expressed in a timely and spatially controlled manner, allowing cells to respond to external cues and maintain homeostasis.

Understanding the regulatory mechanisms that govern gene expression is crucial for engineers seeking to manipulate genes for therapeutic purposes. By deciphering these intricate processes, engineers can develop innovative techniques to modify gene expression patterns, correct genetic abnormalities, and potentially cure genetic diseases.

One of the key components of gene expression regulation is transcription factors. These proteins bind to specific DNA sequences and either activate or repress gene expression. By manipulating the activity of transcription factors, engineers can control the expression of target genes. This knowledge has paved the way for the development of gene editing technologies like CRISPR-Cas9, enabling precise modifications of the genome.

Moreover, epigenetic modifications also play a significant role in gene expression regulation. These modifications, such as DNA methylation and histone acetylation, can alter the accessibility of genes to transcriptional machinery. Engineers can exploit these epigenetic mechanisms to modulate gene expression patterns and potentially reverse aberrant gene silencing associated with diseases like cancer.

Additionally, engineers must understand the role of non-coding RNA molecules in gene expression regulation. MicroRNAs, for example, can bind to messenger RNA molecules and prevent their translation into proteins. Harnessing the potential of these small RNA molecules holds promise in developing targeted therapies for various diseases.

In conclusion, gene expression and regulation are crucial concepts for engineers in the field of biomedical science and biotechnology. A comprehensive understanding of the regulatory mechanisms at play empowers engineers to develop novel genetic engineering and gene therapy techniques. By leveraging transcription factors, epigenetic modifications, and non-coding RNA molecules, engineers can manipulate gene expression patterns, correct genetic abnormalities, and potentially pave the way for groundbreaking advancements in precision medicine.

Chapter 3: Tools and Techniques in Genetic Engineering

Recombinant DNA Technology

Recombinant DNA Technology: Revolutionizing Biomedical Science and Biotechnology

Introduction:
Recombinant DNA technology has emerged as a groundbreaking technique in the field of genetic engineering, offering engineers in the biomedical science and biotechnology niches unparalleled opportunities for innovation and advancement. This subchapter aims to elucidate the principles, techniques, and applications of recombinant DNA technology, equipping engineers with a comprehensive understanding of this transformative field.

1. Understanding Recombinant DNA Technology: Recombinant DNA technology involves the manipulation and combination of DNA molecules from different sources to create new genetic material. This technique allows engineers to isolate, study, and modify specific genes, making it a powerful tool for research and industrial applications.

2. Key Techniques in Recombinant DNA Technology:
a. Gene Cloning: This process involves the insertion of a gene of interest into a vector, such as a plasmid or a bacteriophage, to create a recombinant DNA molecule. The resulting recombinant DNA can then be replicated and propagated in host organisms for further study or industrial production.

b. Polymerase Chain Reaction (PCR): PCR is a technique that amplifies a specific DNA sequence, enabling engineers to produce large quantities of a particular gene or DNA fragment for analysis or manipulation.

c. DNA Sequencing: This technique enables engineers to determine the exact order of nucleotides in a DNA molecule, providing valuable insights into gene structure and function.

3. Applications of Recombinant DNA Technology:
a. Biomedical Research: Recombinant DNA technology has revolutionized the study of genetics, allowing engineers to investigate the causes of diseases, develop diagnostic tests, and explore potential therapeutic interventions.
b. Pharmaceutical Industry: By harnessing recombinant DNA technology, engineers can produce recombinant proteins, such as insulin and growth factors, on a large scale, facilitating the development of novel drugs and biologics.
c. Agriculture and Food Technology: Genetic engineering techniques, including recombinant DNA technology, have been instrumental in developing genetically modified crops with improved traits such as pest resistance and increased nutritional value.
d. Environmental Applications: Recombinant DNA technology offers engineers the tools to address environmental challenges, such as bioremediation, by designing microorganisms capable of degrading pollutants.

Conclusion:
Recombinant DNA technology has revolutionized the fields of biomedical science and biotechnology, empowering engineers to unravel the complexities of genetic information and develop

innovative solutions to pressing challenges. This subchapter has provided a comprehensive overview of the principles, techniques, and applications of recombinant DNA technology, equipping engineers with the knowledge and tools necessary to contribute to the rapidly evolving landscape of genetic engineering and gene therapy.

Polymerase Chain Reaction (PCR)

In the ever-evolving field of biomedical science and biotechnology, Polymerase Chain Reaction (PCR) stands as a vital technique that has revolutionized genetic engineering and gene therapy. As engineers exploring the possibilities of this groundbreaking technology, it is crucial to understand the principles and applications of PCR.

PCR is a technique used to amplify a specific segment of DNA, allowing scientists and researchers to produce a large number of identical copies. This process is achieved through a series of temperature-controlled cycles that involve the denaturation, annealing, and extension of DNA. By utilizing a heat-stable DNA polymerase enzyme, such as Taq polymerase, PCR can replicate DNA segments with high accuracy and efficiency.

The applications of PCR are vast and diverse, spanning numerous fields within biomedical science and biotechnology. In the realm of genetic engineering, PCR plays a crucial role in gene cloning, gene mapping, and DNA sequencing. It enables engineers to isolate and manipulate specific genes, paving the way for advancements in genetic modification and the development of genetically modified organisms (GMOs).

In gene therapy, PCR plays a pivotal role in the diagnosis and treatment of genetic disorders. Scientists can detect specific genetic mutations and variations through PCR-based techniques like allele-specific PCR and real-time PCR. Furthermore, PCR is instrumental in producing therapeutic vectors for gene delivery, facilitating the introduction of healthy genes into patients with genetic diseases.

Understanding the various PCR variants is also essential for engineers in the biomedical science and biotechnology niches. These include reverse transcription PCR (RT-PCR), which allows the amplification of RNA molecules, and quantitative PCR (qPCR), which enables the quantification of DNA or RNA samples. Additionally, multiplex PCR allows the simultaneous amplification of multiple target sequences, while nested PCR enhances the sensitivity and specificity of amplification.

As engineers, it is crucial to stay updated with the latest advancements and techniques in PCR. Innovations such as digital PCR and droplet PCR are pushing the boundaries of this technology, offering higher precision and sensitivity in DNA amplification.

In conclusion, Polymerase Chain Reaction (PCR) is a pivotal technique in genetic engineering and gene therapy. By amplifying specific segments of DNA, engineers can make significant contributions to the fields of biomedical science and biotechnology. As we continue to explore the possibilities of PCR, its applications will undoubtedly expand, driving advancements in precision engineering and shaping the future of genetic research and therapy.

DNA Sequencing and Analysis

In the field of precision engineering, DNA sequencing and analysis play a crucial role in advancing genetic engineering and gene therapy techniques. As engineers, it is essential for us to understand the fundamentals of DNA sequencing and the subsequent analysis methods to design and develop innovative solutions in the fields of biomedical science and biotechnology.

DNA sequencing is the process of determining the precise order of nucleotides within a DNA molecule. This breakthrough technology has revolutionized the way we study genes, genetic variations, and their implications in various diseases. By deciphering the genetic code, engineers can identify mutations, analyze gene expression patterns, and uncover the molecular basis of diseases.

There are several techniques available for DNA sequencing, including Sanger sequencing, next-generation sequencing (NGS), and emerging technologies like nanopore sequencing. Each method has its advantages and limitations, and engineers need to weigh these factors when selecting the appropriate sequencing technology for their applications. Understanding the underlying principles, accuracy, throughput, and cost considerations of these techniques is crucial for effective decision-making.

Once DNA sequencing is completed, the subsequent analysis of the generated data is equally significant. Engineers must be proficient in bioinformatics tools and techniques to interpret the vast amount of sequencing data accurately. This involves aligning sequences, identifying genetic variations, predicting gene function, and analyzing gene expression profiles.

In recent years, the application of DNA sequencing and analysis has extended beyond basic research. It has paved the way for personalized medicine, where an individual's genetic information is used to tailor treatments for specific diseases. Engineers can contribute to this field by developing innovative diagnostic tools, drug delivery systems, and targeted therapies based on DNA sequencing data.

Moreover, DNA sequencing and analysis have become crucial in agriculture, forensics, and environmental studies. These applications have highlighted the interdisciplinary nature of genetic engineering and the importance of collaboration between engineers and experts in other scientific disciplines.

In summary, DNA sequencing and analysis are indispensable tools for engineers working in the fields of biomedical science and biotechnology. By understanding the principles, techniques, and applications of DNA sequencing, engineers can contribute to the development of precision engineering solutions that improve human health, enhance agricultural practices, and protect the environment. As this field continues to evolve rapidly, it is essential for engineers to stay updated with the latest advancements and embrace the interdisciplinary nature of genetic engineering to drive innovation forward.

Gene Cloning and Expression

Gene cloning and expression are fundamental techniques in the field of genetic engineering, which hold immense potential for engineers working in the biomedical science and biotechnology industries. This subchapter aims to provide engineers with a comprehensive understanding of the principles, methods, and applications of gene cloning and expression.

Gene cloning involves the isolation and replication of a specific gene or DNA fragment of interest. This technique allows researchers to study the function and structure of genes, as well as produce large quantities of specific DNA sequences. Various methods, such as polymerase chain reaction (PCR), restriction enzyme digestion, and DNA ligation, are employed during the gene cloning process. Engineers can utilize these techniques to manipulate genetic material and develop new bio-based products, therapies, or diagnostic tools.

Once a gene of interest is cloned, the next step is expression, which involves the production of a desired protein using the cloned gene as a template. Protein expression can be achieved in both prokaryotic and eukaryotic systems, each offering unique advantages and challenges. Prokaryotic expression systems, such as Escherichia coli (E. coli), are simple, cost-effective, and widely used. Eukaryotic expression systems, such as yeast or mammalian cells, are capable of post-translational modifications and produce more complex proteins. Engineers need to consider factors such as gene codon optimization, vector selection, and protein purification methods when designing an expression system for a specific protein.

The applications of gene cloning and expression techniques are vast and diverse. In biomedicine, these techniques play a crucial role in the production of recombinant proteins for therapeutic purposes, such as insulin, growth factors, and antibodies. They also enable the development of gene therapies, where defective genes are replaced with functional ones to treat genetic disorders. In biotechnology, gene cloning and expression are used for the production of enzymes, biofuels, and bioplastics, as well as the engineering of crops with desirable traits.

Engineers working in the biomedical science and biotechnology fields can greatly benefit from understanding and mastering gene cloning and expression techniques. These powerful tools allow for the manipulation and production of genetic material, enabling the development of innovative solutions to pressing challenges in healthcare, agriculture, and environmental sustainability. By harnessing the potential of gene cloning and expression, engineers can contribute to the advancement of precision engineering and the betterment of society as a whole.

Chapter 4: Genetic Engineering Applications in Engineering

Genetic Modification of Microorganisms

In the ever-evolving field of biomedical science and biotechnology, genetic modification of microorganisms has emerged as a powerful tool for engineers. This subchapter delves into the fascinating world of manipulating the genetic makeup of microorganisms to unlock their potential for various applications.

Microorganisms, such as bacteria and yeast, are invaluable in industrial processes, healthcare, and environmental remediation. However, their natural capabilities can be limited, hindering their full potential in addressing complex challenges. Genetic engineering offers a solution by providing engineers with the ability to modify the genetic material of microorganisms, enhancing their functionality and tailoring them to specific needs.

One of the primary applications of genetic modification in microorganisms is the production of therapeutic proteins and vaccines. Engineers can introduce genes encoding the desired protein into the microorganism's genome, allowing it to produce large quantities of the protein efficiently. This technique has revolutionized the production of insulin, human growth hormone, and numerous other biologics, improving the lives of millions.

Furthermore, genetically modified microorganisms can be designed to degrade harmful pollutants or produce valuable chemicals. Through targeted genetic modifications, engineers can enhance the metabolic pathways of microorganisms, enabling them to efficiently break down toxic compounds present in the environment. This approach holds enormous potential for environmental remediation and the development of sustainable biofuels.

The subchapter also explores the ethical considerations surrounding genetic modification of microorganisms. Engineers must navigate the fine line between the benefits and potential risks associated with these technologies. The responsible use of genetically modified microorganisms requires stringent safety precautions to prevent unintended consequences, such as the release of genetically modified organisms into the environment.

Overall, this subchapter provides engineers with a comprehensive understanding of the techniques and applications of genetic modification in microorganisms. It emphasizes the importance of precision engineering in harnessing the full potential of microorganisms, and highlights the role of engineers in driving innovation in biomedical science and biotechnology.

As the field of genetic engineering continues to advance, engineers specializing in biomedical science and biotechnology will play a crucial role in shaping the future of precision engineering. By exploring the genetic modification of microorganisms, engineers can contribute to groundbreaking discoveries and innovations in healthcare, environmental sustainability, and beyond.

Genetic Engineering in Agriculture

Introduction:

The field of genetic engineering has revolutionized various industries, and agriculture is no exception. With the increasing global population and the need for sustainable food production, genetic engineering techniques have become invaluable in improving crop yields, enhancing nutritional content, and developing disease-resistant plants. This subchapter will delve into the applications of genetic engineering in agriculture, highlighting its significance for engineers in the biomedical science and biotechnology niches.

Enhancing Crop Yield:

One of the primary objectives of genetic engineering in agriculture is to enhance crop yield. Through the manipulation of plant genomes, scientists have been able to develop crops with improved growth characteristics, such as increased resistance to pests, diseases, and environmental stresses. Engineers play a crucial role in optimizing these genetic modifications to ensure the desired traits are successfully incorporated into the crops, ultimately leading to higher productivity.

Improving Nutritional Value:

Another area where genetic engineering has made significant contributions is in enhancing the nutritional value of crops. By modifying the genetic makeup of plants, engineers have successfully increased the levels of essential nutrients, such as vitamins and minerals, in various food crops. This has had a profound impact on addressing malnutrition and improving overall human health.

Engineers in the biomedical science and biotechnology fields are at the forefront of designing and implementing these genetic modifications to ensure the safety and efficacy of these nutrient-enriched crops.

Developing Disease-Resistant Plants:

Plant diseases can wreak havoc on agricultural systems, leading to significant crop losses and economic hardships for farmers. Genetic engineering offers a solution by developing disease-resistant plants. Through techniques like gene editing and genetic modification, engineers can introduce genes that confer resistance to specific pathogens. This approach reduces the reliance on chemical pesticides, making agriculture more sustainable and environmentally friendly.

Challenges and Ethical Considerations:

While genetic engineering in agriculture offers immense benefits, it also presents challenges and ethical considerations. Engineers must navigate issues related to intellectual property rights, biosafety regulations, and public acceptance. It is essential for engineers in the biomedical science and biotechnology niches to be well-versed in these matters and contribute to the development of robust ethical frameworks that guide the responsible use of genetic engineering techniques in agriculture.

Conclusion:

Genetic engineering has transformed agriculture, enabling engineers in the biomedical science and biotechnology niches to improve crop yields, enhance nutritional content, and develop disease-resistant plants. As the demand for sustainable food production continues to grow, engineers play a crucial role in optimizing these genetic modifications, ensuring their safety, efficacy, and compliance with ethical considerations. By harnessing the power of genetic engineering, engineers are contributing to a more sustainable and resilient agricultural system that can meet the challenges of the future.

Industrial Applications

In recent years, precision engineering has emerged as a critical tool in the field of industrial applications, particularly in the domains of biomedical science and biotechnology. The integration of genetic engineering and gene therapy techniques has revolutionized the way engineers approach various challenges in these sectors. This subchapter explores the diverse industrial applications of precision engineering, shedding light on its transformative potential for engineers working in the domains of biomedical science and biotechnology.

One of the major areas where precision engineering has made significant advancements is in the development of pharmaceuticals. Engineers have employed genetic engineering techniques to enhance the production of therapeutic proteins, antibodies, and vaccines. By manipulating the genetic makeup of host organisms, such as bacteria and mammalian cells, engineers can optimize their ability to produce high-quality pharmaceutical products. Precision engineering provides the means to modify these organisms at the genetic level, enabling the production of complex molecules that were previously difficult to obtain.

Furthermore, precision engineering has also contributed to the creation of novel diagnostic tools and techniques. Through genetic engineering, engineers can design and develop advanced biosensors capable of detecting specific genetic markers associated with diseases. These biosensors can be utilized for early detection, monitoring disease progression, and assessing treatment efficacy. The precision offered by genetic engineering empowers engineers to create highly sensitive and specific diagnostic tools, revolutionizing the field of medical diagnostics.

In the realm of biotechnology, precision engineering has opened up new avenues for the production of biofuels and biochemicals. By genetically modifying microorganisms, engineers can enhance their ability to convert renewable resources, such as agricultural waste and algae, into valuable products. Precision engineering techniques enable engineers to optimize metabolic pathways and improve the efficiency of bioconversion processes, leading to more sustainable and economically viable solutions.

In conclusion, precision engineering has emerged as a powerful tool in industrial applications, particularly within the domains of biomedical science and biotechnology. By integrating genetic engineering and gene therapy techniques, engineers can push the boundaries of pharmaceutical production, diagnostic tools, and biotechnology applications. The transformative potential of precision engineering lies in its ability to manipulate and optimize genetic material at the molecular level. As engineers continue to explore and refine these techniques, the possibilities for industrial applications in biomedical science and biotechnology are boundless.

Environmental Applications

In recent years, the field of precision engineering has expanded its horizons beyond biomedical science and biotechnology, branching out to address pressing environmental challenges. Engineers have begun to harness the power of genetic engineering and gene therapy techniques to find innovative solutions to environmental issues, contributing to a sustainable and greener future.

One of the most significant applications of precision engineering in the environmental realm is the remediation of contaminated sites. Traditional methods of cleaning up polluted sites, such as landfills or industrial areas, often involve expensive and time-consuming processes. However, with the advent of genetic engineering, engineers are now able to develop organisms capable of breaking down toxic substances and pollutants more efficiently.

By modifying the genetic makeup of microorganisms, engineers can enhance their ability to degrade specific contaminants. These modified organisms, known as bioremediation agents, can be introduced into contaminated sites to accelerate the degradation process. This approach offers a cost-effective and environmentally friendly alternative to traditional remediation methods, reducing the long-term impact of pollutants on ecosystems and human health.

Precision engineering techniques are also being applied to address the global challenge of plastic waste. With millions of tons of plastic entering our oceans and landfills each year, there is an urgent need for innovative solutions. Engineers are now using genetic engineering to develop microorganisms capable of metabolizing and degrading plastic. These engineered microorganisms can break down plastics into harmless byproducts, reducing the environmental burden of plastic waste.

Another exciting application of precision engineering in the environmental sector is the development of genetically modified crops. By incorporating specific genes into crop plants, engineers can enhance their resistance to pests, diseases, and adverse environmental conditions. This not only increases crop yields but also reduces the need for chemical pesticides and fertilizers, minimizing their impact on the environment.

Furthermore, precision engineering techniques are contributing to the development of sustainable biofuels. By engineering microorganisms to produce biofuels from renewable sources, engineers are paving the way for a cleaner and more sustainable energy future. These biofuels can replace fossil fuels, reducing greenhouse gas emissions and dependence on non-renewable resources.

In conclusion, the field of precision engineering is making significant strides in addressing environmental challenges. By applying genetic engineering and gene therapy techniques, engineers are revolutionizing the way we approach pollution remediation, plastic waste management, crop production, and renewable energy. As engineers in the niches of biomedical science and biotechnology, it is crucial to stay updated on the latest developments in environmental applications, as our expertise and innovative solutions are essential for creating a sustainable future.

Chapter 5: Introduction to Gene Therapy

Understanding Gene Therapy

Gene therapy is a groundbreaking field in biomedical science and biotechnology that holds immense potential for revolutionizing the treatment of various genetic disorders. As engineers, it is crucial to have a comprehensive understanding of this cutting-edge technology to contribute effectively to the field of precision engineering.

Gene therapy involves the alteration or modification of specific genes within an individual's cells to treat, prevent, or cure diseases. By introducing therapeutic genes into the body, this technique aims to replace or compensate for faulty or missing genes responsible for genetic disorders. This innovative approach holds promise for treating a wide range of conditions, including inherited disorders, cancer, cardiovascular diseases, and neurodegenerative disorders.

One of the key challenges in gene therapy is delivering the therapeutic genes to the target cells effectively. Engineers play a vital role in developing precise and efficient delivery systems, such as viral vectors or non-viral delivery methods, to ensure successful gene transfer. These delivery systems must navigate the complex biological barriers and deliver the therapeutic genes safely and specifically to the desired cells or tissues.

Understanding the different types of gene therapy is essential for engineers to contribute meaningfully to this field. There are three main approaches to gene therapy: replacing a faulty gene with a functional one, inactivating or suppressing a malfunctioning gene, and introducing new genes to enhance the body's ability to fight diseases. Each approach requires a deep understanding of the specific genetic mechanisms involved and the engineering techniques required for precise gene manipulation.

Moreover, engineers must also be aware of the ethical and safety considerations associated with gene therapy. As this technology continues to evolve, it is crucial to ensure that gene therapies are safe, effective, and ethically sound. Adhering to strict regulatory guidelines, engineers must design gene therapy techniques that minimize potential risks and maximize therapeutic benefits.

In conclusion, understanding gene therapy is of paramount importance for engineers in the fields of biomedical science and biotechnology. By comprehending the underlying principles, delivery systems, and ethical considerations, engineers can contribute to the development of precise and effective gene therapy techniques. This knowledge will enable engineers to collaborate with scientists and medical professionals to advance the field of precision engineering and bring about transformative changes in healthcare.

Types of Gene Therapy

Gene therapy is a rapidly advancing field in biomedicine that holds immense potential for treating a wide range of genetic disorders and diseases. As engineers, it is crucial to understand the various techniques and approaches used in gene therapy to contribute to the development of innovative solutions in the biomedical science and biotechnology industries. This subchapter explores the different types of gene therapy, shedding light on their principles, applications, and challenges.

1. Gene Addition Therapy: This approach involves introducing a functional copy of a gene into the patient's cells to compensate for the defective or missing gene causing the disease. Viral vectors, such as retroviruses and adenoviruses, are commonly used to deliver the therapeutic gene into the target cells. Gene addition therapy shows promise in treating disorders caused by single gene mutations, such as cystic fibrosis and hemophilia.

2. Gene Editing Therapy: Gene editing techniques, like CRISPR-Cas9, have revolutionized the field by enabling precise modifications of the genome. This therapy aims at correcting or modifying the faulty genes responsible for diseases. Engineers play a vital role in optimizing gene editing tools and delivery systems to enhance their efficiency and minimize off-target effects. Gene editing therapy holds great potential in treating genetic disorders like sickle cell anemia and muscular dystrophy.

3. Gene Silencing Therapy: Also known as RNA interference (RNAi), this approach targets the messenger RNA (mRNA) molecules that carry instructions for producing disease-causing proteins. Small interfering RNA (siRNA) molecules are designed to bind to specific mRNA sequences and prevent their translation into proteins. Gene silencing therapy has shown promise in treating conditions like Huntington's disease and amyotrophic lateral sclerosis (ALS).

4. Gene Regulation Therapy: This strategy aims to modulate the expression of specific genes without altering their sequence. Transcription factors or regulatory proteins are used to either activate or suppress the expression of target genes. Gene regulation therapy holds potential in treating complex diseases that involve dysregulated gene expression, such as cancer and metabolic disorders.

While gene therapy offers promising solutions, there are challenges to overcome. Engineers are essential in developing advanced delivery systems, optimizing vectors, and ensuring precise targeting to enhance efficacy and safety. Additionally, addressing ethical considerations, long-term effects, and potential immune responses are crucial aspects of gene therapy research and development.

In conclusion, understanding the different types of gene therapy is essential for engineers working in the fields of biomedical science and biotechnology. Each approach has its unique advantages and challenges, and continuous innovation and collaboration between engineering and medical disciplines are crucial in advancing the field of gene therapy for the benefit of patients worldwide.

Challenges and Ethical Considerations in Gene Therapy

In recent years, gene therapy has emerged as a groundbreaking field with immense potential for revolutionizing the treatment of genetic disorders. This subchapter aims to delve into the challenges and ethical considerations that engineers working in the biomedical science and biotechnology niches may encounter in the development and implementation of gene therapy techniques.

One of the primary challenges faced by engineers in gene therapy is the delivery of therapeutic genes into target cells effectively. This process, known as gene delivery, requires efficient methods to transport the therapeutic genes into the desired cells while avoiding immune system responses and potential off-target effects. Engineers are tasked with developing innovative delivery systems such as viral vectors, nanoparticles, liposomes, and electroporation techniques to enhance the efficiency and safety of gene delivery.

Another significant challenge lies in the precise editing of the genome without causing unintended mutations or disruptions. Advances in gene editing technologies like CRISPR-Cas9 have opened up new possibilities for gene therapy, but engineers must ensure the accuracy and specificity of these tools to avoid potential side effects or ethical concerns. The ethical considerations surrounding gene editing are particularly crucial, as the ability to manipulate the human genome raises questions about the boundaries of human enhancement and the potential for eugenic applications.

Furthermore, the long-term effects and safety of gene therapy must be carefully evaluated. Engineers must conduct extensive preclinical and clinical trials to assess the efficacy and safety of gene therapy techniques. This involves monitoring potential adverse effects, detecting any immunogenic responses, and determining the durability of therapeutic effects over time. The interdisciplinary collaboration between engineers, biologists, clinicians, and regulatory bodies is essential to address these challenges and ensure the successful translation of gene therapy techniques from the laboratory to clinical practice.

Ethical considerations play a pivotal role in gene therapy, as engineers must navigate the complex landscape of genetic manipulation. Issues such as patient autonomy, consent, equitable access, and the potential for genetic discrimination require careful deliberation and adherence to ethical guidelines. Engineers must prioritize the principles of beneficence, non-maleficence, autonomy, and justice to ensure that gene therapy is employed responsibly and for the benefit of patients.

In conclusion, gene therapy holds immense promise for addressing genetic disorders, but engineers working in the biomedical science and biotechnology niches must overcome various challenges and ethical considerations. By focusing on optimizing gene delivery, enhancing precision in gene editing, evaluating long-term safety, and adhering to ethical guidelines, engineers can contribute to the advancement of gene therapy techniques and their responsible implementation in clinical settings.

Chapter 6: Gene Delivery Systems

Viral Vectors

Viral Vectors: Revolutionizing Genetic Engineering and Gene Therapy Techniques for Engineers

Introduction:

In the field of biomedical science and biotechnology, engineers play a crucial role in developing innovative techniques to improve human health. One such breakthrough is the use of viral vectors in genetic engineering and gene therapy. Viral vectors have revolutionized the field, offering a promising approach to deliver therapeutic genes to target cells and restore normal cellular function. This subchapter aims to provide engineers with a comprehensive understanding of viral vectors and their applications in precision engineering.

Understanding Viral Vectors:

Viral vectors are genetically modified viruses that act as delivery vehicles to transfer specific genes into target cells. These viruses have been engineered to remove their disease-causing properties while retaining their ability to enter cells efficiently. The most commonly used viral vectors include adenoviruses, lentiviruses, retroviruses, and adeno-associated viruses (AAVs). Each viral vector has unique characteristics and is tailored for specific applications.

Applications in Genetic Engineering:

Engineers have harnessed the potential of viral vectors to introduce new genes into cells for various purposes. Genetic engineering with viral vectors has paved the way for the production of recombinant proteins, such as insulin, in large quantities for therapeutic purposes. Additionally, viral vectors have been instrumental in developing gene editing technologies like CRISPR-Cas9, enabling precise modifications to the genome.

Gene Therapy Techniques:

Viral vectors have emerged as a powerful tool in gene therapy, a revolutionary approach to treat genetic disorders and other diseases. By delivering therapeutic genes into target cells, viral vectors can correct genetic defects, restore normal cellular function, and potentially cure previously incurable diseases. Gene therapies using viral vectors have shown promising results in treating conditions like cystic fibrosis, hemophilia, and certain types of cancer.

Engineering Challenges and Advancements:

While viral vectors offer immense potential, engineers face several challenges in their development and application. These challenges include vector stability, immune response, and the need for improved targeting and safety profiles. However, researchers and engineers are constantly striving to address these challenges through advancements in vector design, molecular engineering, and gene delivery techniques.

Conclusion:

Viral vectors have revolutionized genetic engineering and gene therapy techniques, offering immense potential for engineers in the fields of biomedical science and biotechnology. By understanding the fundamentals of viral vectors and their applications, engineers can contribute significantly to the development of precise and effective genetic therapies. As the field continues to advance, engineers will play a crucial role in overcoming challenges and unlocking the full potential of viral vectors, ultimately improving the lives of countless individuals affected by genetic disorders and diseases.

Non-viral Vectors

In the field of genetic engineering and gene therapy, vectors play a crucial role in the delivery of therapeutic genes into target cells. While viral vectors have been extensively used for this purpose, non-viral vectors offer a promising alternative with several advantages. This subchapter aims to introduce engineers to the concept of non-viral vectors and their applications in precision engineering within the fields of biomedical science and biotechnology.

Non-viral vectors are synthetic delivery systems that can transport therapeutic genes into cells without the use of viral components. They are typically composed of nucleic acid molecules, such as plasmid DNA or mRNA, encapsulated within various materials, including lipids, polymers, and nanoparticles. The development of non-viral vectors has revolutionized gene therapy by addressing some of the limitations associated with viral vectors, such as safety concerns, immunogenicity, and limited cargo capacity.

One major advantage of non-viral vectors is their enhanced safety profile. Unlike viral vectors, which can trigger immune responses and potentially lead to adverse effects, non-viral vectors are generally well-tolerated by the body. This makes them ideal for long-term applications, where multiple administrations may be required. Additionally, non-viral vectors can accommodate larger genetic payloads, allowing for the delivery of multiple therapeutic genes simultaneously, which is crucial for complex diseases with multifactorial origins.

Engineers in the field of biomedical science and biotechnology can harness the potential of non-viral vectors to overcome specific challenges. For instance, the ability to modify and optimize the vector formulation allows for precise control over the delivery process. By engineering the size, charge, and surface properties of the vector particles, engineers can enhance cellular uptake, target specific tissues or cells, and regulate gene expression levels.

Moreover, non-viral vectors offer versatility and scalability, making them suitable for various applications in gene therapy. They can be administered via different routes, including intravenous, intramuscular, or local injections, as well as through inhalation or topical application. This flexibility allows for the development of tailored gene therapies for diverse diseases, including genetic disorders, cancer, cardiovascular diseases, and neurological disorders.

In summary, non-viral vectors present a promising avenue for precision engineering in the fields of biomedical science and biotechnology. With their improved safety profile, larger cargo capacity, and customizable properties, non-viral vectors offer a versatile and efficient platform for the delivery of therapeutic genes. Engineers have the opportunity to contribute to the development and optimization of these vectors, paving the way for innovative gene therapies that can revolutionize the treatment of complex diseases.

Advancements in Gene Delivery Systems

In recent years, the field of genetic engineering has witnessed remarkable progress, largely due to significant advancements in gene delivery systems. These systems play a crucial role in the successful transfer of genetic material into target cells, enabling engineers to manipulate and modify the genetic makeup of various organisms for therapeutic purposes. This subchapter provides an overview of the latest breakthroughs in gene delivery systems and their implications for the fields of biomedical science and biotechnology.

One of the most notable advancements in gene delivery systems is the development of viral vectors. Viruses have evolved sophisticated mechanisms to deliver their genetic material into host cells, making them an ideal tool for gene transfer. By modifying viral genomes, engineers can create safe and efficient viral vectors that can selectively deliver therapeutic genes to specific cells or tissues. These advancements have paved the way for gene therapy, a promising approach that harnesses the power of gene delivery systems to treat genetic disorders and chronic diseases.

Non-viral gene delivery systems have also seen significant advancements. Unlike viral vectors, non-viral systems do not rely on viral components and offer several advantages, including reduced immunogenicity and improved safety profiles. Researchers have developed various non-viral delivery systems, such as liposomes, nanoparticles, and gene guns, each with unique properties and mechanisms of action. These systems have expanded the possibilities of gene therapy by enabling the delivery of genes to previously inaccessible tissues and organs.

Furthermore, advancements in gene delivery systems have revolutionized the field of genome editing. Techniques such as CRISPR-Cas9 have emerged as powerful tools for precise genetic modifications. Gene delivery systems, including viral vectors and nanoparticles, play a crucial role in delivering CRISPR components into target cells, allowing engineers to edit genes with unprecedented accuracy and efficiency. This breakthrough has opened up new avenues for addressing genetic diseases and developing personalized medicine approaches.

The advancements in gene delivery systems have not only accelerated research in the biomedical sciences but also have implications for biotechnology. Gene delivery systems have enabled the production of recombinant proteins, biofuels, and industrial enzymes by introducing genes into microbial hosts or plant cells. These systems have revolutionized the production processes, making them more efficient and cost-effective.

In conclusion, advancements in gene delivery systems have revolutionized the field of genetic engineering, offering new possibilities for engineers in the biomedical science and biotechnology niches. The development of viral and non-viral vectors, as well as their applications in gene therapy and genome editing, have paved the way for innovative treatments and personalized medicine approaches. Additionally, gene delivery systems have transformed the biotechnology industry by facilitating the production of valuable compounds and bio-based products. As engineers continue to refine gene delivery systems, the potential for precision engineering in genetic engineering and gene therapy techniques is boundless.

Chapter 7: Gene Editing Techniques

CRISPR-Cas9 System

The CRISPR-Cas9 system has revolutionized the field of genetic engineering and gene therapy, offering engineers in the biomedical science and biotechnology niches an unprecedented tool for precise genome editing. This subchapter provides engineers with a comprehensive understanding of the CRISPR-Cas9 system, its underlying mechanisms, and its applications in various fields.

The CRISPR-Cas9 system is a powerful gene editing tool derived from the natural immune system of bacteria. CRISPR stands for Clustered Regularly Interspaced Short Palindromic Repeats, which are segments of DNA that contain short repetitions of base sequences. These repeats act as a defense mechanism against viral infections, as they allow the bacteria to recognize and destroy foreign DNA.

The Cas9 enzyme, on the other hand, is a protein that acts as a pair of molecular "scissors." It can precisely cut DNA at specific locations, guided by a small RNA molecule called the guide RNA (gRNA). By introducing a customized gRNA, scientists can direct Cas9 to any desired location in the genome, enabling them to edit or modify specific genes with unparalleled precision.

The applications of the CRISPR-Cas9 system are vast and diverse. In the field of biomedicine, it has the potential to treat genetic disorders by correcting disease-causing mutations. Engineers can utilize this system to develop new gene therapies, providing hope for patients suffering from previously incurable conditions.

In agriculture, the CRISPR-Cas9 system offers a way to improve crop yields, enhance disease resistance, and increase nutritional value. By precisely editing the genes responsible for certain traits, engineers can create crops that are more resilient to environmental challenges and capable of addressing food shortages.

Furthermore, the CRISPR-Cas9 system has also revolutionized the field of basic research. Its ease of use and low cost have made it accessible to a wide range of scientists, enabling breakthrough discoveries in various disciplines, from understanding the fundamental mechanisms of diseases to studying the intricacies of embryonic development.

However, the CRISPR-Cas9 system also raises ethical considerations. The potential for editing human embryos or germline cells sparks debates on the moral implications and long-term consequences. Engineers must be aware of the ethical guidelines and regulations governing the use of this technology to ensure responsible and ethical application.

In conclusion, the CRISPR-Cas9 system is a groundbreaking tool that holds immense potential for engineers in the biomedical science and biotechnology fields. Its ability to precisely edit genes offers unprecedented opportunities for disease treatment, crop improvement, and scientific discoveries. However, it is essential for engineers to approach this technology with ethical considerations, ensuring its responsible and beneficial application for the betterment of society.

Zinc Finger Nucleases (ZFNs)

Zinc Finger Nucleases (ZFNs) are a powerful tool in the field of genetic engineering and gene therapy, which holds immense potential for engineers working in the biomedical science and biotechnology niches. This subchapter aims to provide engineers with a comprehensive understanding of ZFNs and their applications in precision engineering.

ZFNs are engineered proteins that can be used to manipulate the DNA sequence in a targeted manner. They consist of a DNA-binding domain called zinc fingers, which can recognize specific DNA sequences, and a DNA-cleavage domain that can induce double-strand breaks (DSBs) at these targeted sites. The ability to precisely target and modify specific genes makes ZFNs an invaluable tool in genetic engineering.

One of the primary applications of ZFNs is in the field of gene therapy. By using ZFNs to induce DSBs at specific sites in the genome, engineers can effectively edit or modify genes responsible for diseases. This precise gene editing holds immense promise for treating genetic disorders such as cystic fibrosis, sickle cell anemia, and Huntington's disease. Engineers can design and construct ZFNs to target the faulty genes, enabling precise correction or elimination of the disease-causing mutations.

Furthermore, ZFNs can also be used for gene knockout studies to understand gene function and identify potential drug targets. By inducing DSBs in specific genes, engineers can disrupt their function and observe the resulting phenotype, providing valuable insights into gene function and disease mechanisms. This information can then be utilized to develop novel therapies or drugs targeting these genes.

Although ZFNs are a powerful tool, their design and construction can be complex. Engineers need to carefully select and design the zinc finger domains to ensure specific and efficient DNA binding. Additionally, optimizing the DNA-cleavage domain is crucial to minimize off-target effects and maximize on-target cleavage.

In conclusion, Zinc Finger Nucleases (ZFNs) are a revolutionary tool in precision genetic engineering. They provide engineers with the ability to precisely target and modify genes, making them invaluable in the fields of gene therapy and gene function studies. By harnessing the power of ZFNs, engineers can contribute to advancements in biomedical science and biotechnology, bringing us closer to effective treatments for genetic diseases and a deeper understanding of the genetic basis of various conditions.

Transcription Activator-Like Effector Nucleases (TALENs)

In recent years, the field of genetic engineering has witnessed significant advancements, leading to the development of powerful tools and techniques that have revolutionized various industries, including biomedical science and biotechnology. One such tool that has gained considerable attention is Transcription Activator-Like Effector Nucleases (TALENs). This subchapter aims to provide engineers with an insight into TALENs and their applications in precision engineering.

TALENs are programmable nucleases derived from naturally occurring transcription activator-like effectors (TALEs) found in certain bacteria. These nucleases have the ability to target specific DNA sequences with incredible precision, making them invaluable tools for genetic manipulation. Unlike other nucleases, TALENs can be tailored to recognize virtually any DNA sequence of interest, allowing researchers to edit genes with unparalleled accuracy.

The applications of TALENs are vast and diverse. In the field of biomedicine, they hold immense potential for the treatment of genetic diseases. By using TALENs to precisely edit disease-causing genes, scientists can potentially correct genetic mutations and alleviate the symptoms of various inherited disorders. This approach, known as gene therapy, has shown promising results in preclinical and clinical trials, offering hope for patients suffering from previously untreatable conditions.

TALENs also find applications in biotechnology, particularly in the development of genetically modified organisms (GMOs) and the production of valuable bioproducts. Through TALEN-mediated genome editing, scientists can introduce desirable traits into plants and animals, improving crop yields, enhancing disease resistance, and even engineering animals to produce therapeutic proteins in their milk or eggs. These advancements have the potential to address global challenges such as food security and the production of life-saving drugs.

Engineers play a crucial role in the development and optimization of TALEN-based technologies. They contribute by designing and constructing TALEN vectors, which are the DNA sequences used to guide the nucleases to their target sites. Additionally, engineers are involved in the development of delivery systems, such as viral vectors or nanoparticles, to efficiently introduce TALENs into target cells.

However, despite their tremendous potential, TALENs still face certain limitations, including off-target effects and the complexity of their design. Researchers are continuously working to improve these nucleases and develop even more precise and efficient tools for genetic engineering.

In conclusion, TALENs represent a remarkable breakthrough in genetic engineering, enabling scientists to manipulate DNA with unprecedented precision. Their applications in biomedicine and biotechnology are vast, offering new possibilities for disease treatment, agriculture, and the production of valuable bioproducts. As engineers, understanding and harnessing the power of TALENs is essential for advancing the field of precision engineering and driving innovation in biomedical science and biotechnology.

Chapter 8: Applications of Gene Therapy in Engineering

Gene Therapy for Genetic Disorders

Gene therapy is a groundbreaking field of research that holds immense potential for the treatment and prevention of genetic disorders. As engineers, our role in this field is crucial as we explore and develop advanced techniques to harness the power of genetic engineering for biomedical science and biotechnology.

Genetic disorders are caused by mutations or abnormalities in our DNA, which can lead to various health conditions such as cystic fibrosis, muscular dystrophy, and sickle cell anemia. Traditional treatments for these disorders focus on managing symptoms rather than addressing the underlying cause. However, gene therapy offers a promising alternative by directly targeting and correcting the faulty genes responsible for these conditions.

One of the key approaches in gene therapy is the delivery of functional genes into the patient's cells. This can be achieved using viral vectors or non-viral methods such as nanoparticles. As engineers, we play a critical role in designing and optimizing these delivery systems to ensure efficient and safe gene transfer. This involves developing novel materials, optimizing particle size and surface properties, and enhancing the stability and targeting ability of the vectors.

Another important aspect of gene therapy is gene editing. Technologies such as CRISPR-Cas9 have revolutionized the field by enabling precise and efficient editing of the genome. As engineers, we can contribute by refining these gene editing tools, improving their accuracy, and exploring new delivery methods to ensure their effective application in clinical settings.

Furthermore, the success of gene therapy relies on our ability to understand and manipulate the complex biological processes involved. This requires interdisciplinary collaboration between engineers and biologists to unravel the intricate mechanisms of gene expression, regulation, and function. By leveraging our engineering expertise, we can develop innovative tools and techniques to study and manipulate genes, paving the way for more effective gene therapy strategies.

In this subchapter, we will delve into the principles and techniques of gene therapy for genetic disorders. We will explore the challenges and opportunities in delivering therapeutic genes, enhancing gene editing technologies, and understanding the underlying biology. By harnessing the power of genetic engineering, we can revolutionize the field of precision medicine and pave the way for personalized therapies tailored to individual patients.

As engineers working in the fields of biomedical science and biotechnology, our expertise is essential in advancing gene therapy techniques and bringing them closer to clinical application. Together, let us embark on this exciting journey of precision engineering and contribute to the development of innovative solutions for genetic disorders.

Gene Therapy for Cancer

Cancer continues to be a major health concern worldwide, with millions of lives affected by this devastating disease. Traditional treatment options, such as chemotherapy and radiation therapy, often come with significant side effects and limited effectiveness. However, recent advancements in genetic engineering and gene therapy techniques offer a promising new approach to combat cancer.

This subchapter will delve into the fascinating field of gene therapy for cancer, specifically addressing engineers who specialize in biomedical science and biotechnology. It aims to provide an overview of the principles, techniques, and potential applications of gene therapy in the fight against cancer.

Gene therapy involves the introduction of genetic material into cancer cells to modify their behavior and restore normal cellular function. The fundamental concept behind gene therapy for cancer is to either correct the genetic abnormalities that contribute to cancer development or enhance the immune system's ability to recognize and eliminate cancer cells.

Several gene therapy techniques have been developed, including viral and non-viral vectors, gene editing tools like CRISPR-Cas9, and gene delivery systems. Engineers play a critical role in designing and optimizing these delivery systems to ensure safe and efficient gene transfer.

The subchapter will explore the different strategies employed in gene therapy for cancer, such as gene replacement therapy, gene inhibition therapy, and immunogene therapy. It will highlight specific examples of successful gene therapy trials and their outcomes, emphasizing the potential for personalized medicine and targeted therapies.

Moreover, the subchapter will discuss the challenges and limitations associated with gene therapy for cancer. These may include immune responses to viral vectors, off-target effects of gene editing tools, and the need for efficient gene delivery to specific tumor sites. Engineers in the biomedical science and biotechnology fields can contribute to overcoming these challenges by developing innovative and sophisticated gene delivery systems and improving the safety and efficacy of gene therapy techniques.

In conclusion, gene therapy holds great promise in the field of cancer treatment. This subchapter serves as a comprehensive introduction to gene therapy for cancer, providing engineers with a solid foundation in the principles and techniques of this exciting field. By fostering interdisciplinary collaboration and innovation, engineers can contribute to advancing gene therapy as a powerful tool in the fight against cancer, ultimately leading to improved patient outcomes and a brighter future in cancer treatment.

Gene Therapy in Tissue Engineering

Gene therapy is a groundbreaking field within tissue engineering that holds immense potential for engineers in the biomedical science and biotechnology niches. This subchapter explores the intersection of gene therapy and tissue engineering, highlighting the innovative techniques and applications that can revolutionize the way we approach regenerative medicine.

Tissue engineering aims to create functional tissues and organs that can replace or repair damaged ones. It involves combining cells, biomaterials, and biochemical factors to generate constructs that mimic the native tissue's structure and function. Gene therapy, on the other hand, involves the introduction, deletion, or modification of genes within an individual's cells to treat or prevent disease.

The integration of gene therapy into tissue engineering brings several advantages. By genetically modifying cells, engineers can enhance their regenerative capabilities, making them more effective at repairing damaged tissues. For example, researchers have successfully used gene therapy to promote the growth of blood vessels in engineered tissues, ensuring sufficient oxygen and nutrient supply.

Gene therapy can also be used to improve the survival and integration of transplanted tissues. By delivering genes that suppress the immune response, engineers can prevent rejection and promote tissue acceptance. Moreover, the ability to modify genes opens up the possibility of personalized medicine, where therapies can be tailored to an individual's unique genetic profile.

This subchapter delves into the various gene therapy techniques that can be employed in tissue engineering. It discusses viral and non-viral vectors for gene delivery, highlighting their advantages and limitations. Additionally, it explores the importance of gene regulation and control systems to ensure the precise expression of therapeutic genes.

Furthermore, the subchapter delves into the challenges and ethical considerations that engineers need to address when working with gene therapy in tissue engineering. It emphasizes the importance of safety, efficacy, and long-term effects to ensure the responsible translation of these technologies into clinical applications.

Overall, gene therapy in tissue engineering represents a frontier that engineers in the biomedical science and biotechnology niches cannot afford to ignore. This subchapter equips them with the knowledge and insights needed to leverage gene therapy techniques in their pursuit of developing innovative regenerative therapies.

Future Possibilities and Innovations in Gene Therapy

Gene therapy has emerged as a promising field in biomedical science and biotechnology, offering a revolutionary approach to treating genetic disorders and diseases. As engineers, it is crucial to understand the future possibilities and innovations in gene therapy to contribute to the development of more precise and effective techniques. This subchapter aims to explore some of the groundbreaking advancements and potential applications that lie ahead.

One of the future possibilities in gene therapy is the development of personalized medicine. As engineers, we can contribute to the design and implementation of precision engineering techniques that enable tailored therapies for individual patients. Through advancements in gene editing tools like CRISPR-Cas9, it is becoming increasingly feasible to correct disease-causing mutations at the genetic level. This personalized approach holds immense potential for treating a wide range of genetic disorders, including cancer, cardiovascular diseases, and inherited conditions.

Additionally, the integration of gene therapy with other emerging technologies is expected to yield remarkable results. For instance, nanotechnology can enhance targeted gene delivery systems, allowing for more precise and efficient delivery of therapeutic genes to specific cells or tissues. As engineers, we can contribute to the development of nanoscale devices and vehicles that can navigate the complexities of the human body, delivering gene therapies with utmost accuracy.

The future of gene therapy also holds promise in the realm of regenerative medicine. By harnessing the potential of stem cells and gene editing technologies, scientists are exploring ways to repair and regenerate damaged tissues and organs. This could revolutionize the treatment of conditions such as spinal cord injuries, diabetes, and neurodegenerative disorders. As engineers, we can play a pivotal role in developing scaffolds, bioreactors, and tissue engineering techniques that facilitate the growth and integration of genetically modified cells and tissues.

Furthermore, advancements in gene therapy may pave the way for the prevention of genetic diseases altogether. Through germline gene therapy, it may be possible to introduce therapeutic genes into reproductive cells, thus ensuring that future generations are not affected by inherited conditions. However, ethical considerations and regulatory frameworks must be carefully addressed before such interventions can be widely implemented.

In conclusion, the future possibilities and innovations in gene therapy hold tremendous potential for transforming healthcare and improving the lives of countless individuals. As engineers, we have the opportunity to contribute to this field by developing precision engineering techniques, integrating gene therapy with other emerging technologies, advancing regenerative medicine, and exploring preventive approaches. By embracing these future possibilities, we can make significant strides towards a future where genetic disorders and diseases are effectively treated and even prevented.

Chapter 9: Regulatory and Safety Considerations in Genetic Engineering and Gene Therapy

Ethical Guidelines for Genetic Engineering

In recent years, genetic engineering has emerged as a powerful tool with immense potential for advancements in the fields of biomedical science and biotechnology. As engineers working in these domains, it is crucial to approach genetic engineering with a strong sense of responsibility and adhere to ethical guidelines to ensure the safety and well-being of individuals and society as a whole. This subchapter aims to outline the key ethical considerations in genetic engineering and provide guidance for engineers to navigate this rapidly evolving field.

First and foremost, engineers must prioritize the principle of informed consent. This means that individuals undergoing genetic engineering procedures should have a clear understanding of the potential risks, benefits, and long-term consequences associated with the interventions. It is vital to obtain explicit consent from patients or research subjects, ensuring they are well-informed and have the autonomy to make decisions about their genetic makeup.

Another critical ethical guideline is the principle of non-maleficence, which emphasizes the obligation to do no harm. Engineers must ensure that any genetic modifications or interventions are thoroughly tested and proven safe before implementation. Rigorous testing and adherence to established safety standards are crucial to minimize the risk of unintended consequences, such as off-target effects or unforeseen health complications.

Equity and justice should also be integral to the ethical framework of genetic engineering. Engineers must strive to promote equal access to genetic therapies and avoid exacerbating existing social inequalities. It is essential to be mindful of potential discrimination and stigmatization resulting from genetic interventions, and to work towards fair distribution and affordability of these technologies.

Transparency and openness are key principles that should guide genetic engineering practices. Engineers should be transparent about their methodologies, findings, and any conflicts of interest. Open communication with stakeholders, including patients, regulatory bodies, and the wider public, fosters trust and ensures accountability in the field.

Lastly, ethical guidelines must encompass rigorous oversight and regulation. Engineers should actively engage with regulatory bodies and adhere to established standards and guidelines. Regular evaluation and monitoring of genetic engineering practices are necessary to ensure ongoing compliance and to address any emerging ethical concerns.

In conclusion, genetic engineering holds great promise for the fields of biomedical science and biotechnology. However, as engineers, it is our responsibility to approach this technology with a strong ethical framework. By prioritizing informed consent, non-maleficence, equity, transparency, and regulation, we can navigate genetic engineering safely and ethically, accelerating progress while protecting the interests of individuals and society as a whole.

Regulatory Bodies and Approval Processes

In the rapidly evolving field of precision engineering, where genetic engineering and gene therapy techniques are being harnessed for groundbreaking advancements, it is crucial for engineers to have a comprehensive understanding of the regulatory bodies and approval processes that govern these technologies. In this subchapter, we will delve into the key regulatory bodies involved in overseeing the development, testing, and implementation of genetic engineering and gene therapy techniques.

The field of precision engineering operates within a complex framework of regulations and guidelines set forth by various organizations. One of the most prominent regulatory bodies is the Food and Drug Administration (FDA) in the United States. The FDA plays a critical role in ensuring the safety and efficacy of precision engineering technologies, particularly those intended for medical applications. Engineers need to be familiar with the FDA's rigorous approval processes, including preclinical testing, Investigational New Drug (IND) applications, and the New Drug Application (NDA) process.

Another important regulatory body is the European Medicines Agency (EMA), which oversees the approval and regulation of precision engineering technologies in Europe. Engineers working in the biotechnology and biomedical science niches must be aware of the EMA's guidelines and requirements for clinical trials, marketing authorization, and post-approval surveillance.

Furthermore, the subchapter will explore other global regulatory bodies, such as the Pharmaceuticals and Medical Devices Agency (PMDA) in Japan, the Therapeutic Goods Administration (TGA) in Australia, and the World Health Organization (WHO). Engineers must understand the specific requirements and processes mandated by these organizations to ensure the safe and ethical development and implementation of precision engineering technologies.

Additionally, the subchapter will provide insights into the ethical considerations and societal implications surrounding regulatory bodies and approval processes. Engineers must be conscious of the moral and ethical aspects of their work, considering factors such as patient safety, privacy, and informed consent.

Understanding the regulatory landscape is vital for engineers in the biotechnology and biomedical science niches, as it influences the development, commercialization, and adoption of precision engineering techniques. By familiarizing themselves with the various regulatory bodies and approval processes, engineers can navigate the complex regulatory environment and contribute to the advancement of genetic engineering and gene therapy techniques in a responsible and compliant manner.

In conclusion, the subchapter "Regulatory Bodies and Approval Processes" provides engineers in the fields of biotechnology and biomedical science with a comprehensive overview of the key regulatory bodies and approval processes that govern precision engineering technologies. By understanding these regulations and guidelines, engineers can ensure the safe, effective, and ethical development and implementation of genetic engineering and gene therapy techniques for the betterment of society.

Safety Measures and Risk Assessment

In the field of precision engineering, the pursuit of excellence and innovation is closely intertwined with the need for safety and risk assessment. As engineers, it is essential to prioritize the well-being of individuals and the environment when working with genetic engineering and gene therapy techniques. This subchapter aims to provide a comprehensive understanding of the safety measures and risk assessment protocols required in the domains of biomedical science and biotechnology.

1. Introduction to Safety Measures
In this section, we will delve into the importance of safety measures and highlight their significance in precision engineering. We will discuss the regulatory framework and guidelines set forth by relevant authorities to ensure the safe implementation of genetic engineering and gene therapy techniques.

2. Risk Assessment in Biomedical Science
Understanding and mitigating risks is crucial during the development and application of precision engineering techniques. This section will explore the process of risk assessment, including hazard identification, risk analysis, and risk evaluation. We will emphasize the need for engineers to identify potential risks, assess their severity and probability, and make informed decisions to minimize the associated hazards.

3. Biosafety Levels and Containment Strategies
Biomedical science and biotechnology laboratories require appropriate containment strategies to ensure the safety of personnel, the

environment, and the general public. This section will introduce the concept of biosafety levels and their relevance in different laboratory settings. We will discuss the specific containment measures and engineering controls required for each level, including personal protective equipment, facility design, and waste management.

4. Training and Standard Operating Procedures
Engineers and scientists working in precision engineering must be equipped with the necessary skills and knowledge to execute their tasks safely. This section will address the importance of training programs and the development of standard operating procedures (SOPs). We will highlight the need for regular training sessions, emergency response drills, and SOPs that outline safe working practices, equipment handling, and waste disposal protocols.

5. Ethical Considerations and Regulatory Compliance
Precision engineering techniques in genetic engineering and gene therapy often raise ethical concerns. This section will explore the ethical considerations associated with these technologies, emphasizing the importance of informed consent, privacy, and equitable access. Additionally, we will elaborate on the regulatory landscape and the need for engineers to comply with ethical guidelines and legal requirements.

By thoroughly understanding safety measures and risk assessment protocols, engineers in the fields of biomedical science and biotechnology can ensure the responsible development and application of precision engineering techniques. Prioritizing safety is not only crucial for the well-being of individuals and the environment but also fundamental for fostering public trust in these innovative technologies.

Chapter 10: Case Studies and Success Stories in Genetic Engineering and Gene Therapy

Case Study 1: Successful Gene Therapy Treatment

Introduction:

In this subchapter, we delve into a remarkable case study that highlights the groundbreaking success of gene therapy treatment. As engineers specializing in biomedical science and biotechnology, it is crucial to understand the potential of genetic engineering and gene therapy techniques. This case study serves as an inspiring example of how precision engineering has revolutionized the field of medicine, offering new hope for patients suffering from genetic disorders.

The Case Study:

The case revolves around a young patient named Sarah, a 10-year-old girl diagnosed with a rare genetic disorder known as muscular dystrophy. Muscular dystrophy is a debilitating condition that weakens the muscles over time, severely limiting mobility and impacting the overall quality of life. Sarah's condition had progressively worsened, leaving her wheelchair-bound and dependent on others for her daily activities.

Approach and Precision Engineering Techniques:

Gene therapy, an emerging field in precision engineering, provided a glimmer of hope for Sarah and her family. The researchers and engineers embarked on a mission to correct the faulty gene responsible for Sarah's muscular dystrophy. They designed a vector, a delivery system capable of delivering the correct gene to the targeted cells within Sarah's body. The vector was engineered to be safe, efficient, and able to penetrate the affected muscle cells.

The team employed several precision engineering techniques to optimize the vector's performance. They utilized advanced genetic engineering tools to precisely insert the corrected gene into the vector, ensuring its stability and functionality. The vector was further modified to enhance its ability to enter the muscle cells, allowing the corrected gene to replace the faulty one.

Successful Treatment and Outcomes:

After extensive preclinical testing, the team administered the vector carrying the corrected gene to Sarah through a minimally invasive procedure. Over the following weeks and months, Sarah's condition began to improve gradually. She regained muscle strength and mobility, allowing her to walk independently for the first time in years.

The success of Sarah's treatment paved the way for further research and development in gene therapy techniques. Today, precision engineers and biomedical scientists continue to refine and expand these techniques, offering hope to countless individuals suffering from genetic disorders.

Conclusion:

This case study serves as a testament to the immense potential of gene therapy in treating genetic disorders. As engineers specializing in biomedical science and biotechnology, it is crucial to stay updated with the latest developments in precision engineering techniques. By harnessing the power of genetic engineering, precision engineers can play a pivotal role in transforming lives and revolutionizing the field of medicine. The successful treatment of Sarah's muscular dystrophy is just the beginning of a new era in precision engineering, promising a brighter future for patients and their families.

Case Study 2: Genetic Engineering Breakthrough in Engineering Field

In the ever-evolving field of engineering, genetic engineering has emerged as a groundbreaking technique with immense potential in various industries, particularly in the realms of biomedical science and biotechnology. This chapter presents an intriguing case study that highlights a remarkable genetic engineering breakthrough, demonstrating the power of this technology to revolutionize the engineering field.

The case study revolves around a team of engineers and scientists who collaborated to develop an innovative gene therapy technique targeting a rare genetic disorder called Duchenne muscular dystrophy (DMD). DMD is a debilitating condition characterized by progressive muscle degeneration, primarily affecting young boys. Traditional treatments have been limited in their effectiveness, prompting the need for a novel approach.

Through meticulous research and experimentation, the team of engineers successfully engineered a viral vector capable of delivering a functional copy of the dystrophin gene – the gene responsible for DMD – into the affected muscle cells. This breakthrough technique utilized the principles of precision engineering to design a highly efficient and targeted delivery system.

The engineers meticulously optimized the viral vector, ensuring its safety and efficacy in delivering the therapeutic gene to the affected cells without triggering any adverse side effects. This required a deep understanding of genetic engineering principles, as well as expertise in bioinformatics, molecular biology, and advanced imaging techniques.

The results were nothing short of extraordinary. In preclinical trials, the engineered viral vector successfully delivered the functional dystrophin gene to the muscle cells of animal models with DMD, resulting in a significant improvement in muscle strength and function. These promising outcomes have paved the way for the translation of this gene therapy technique into clinical trials, offering hope for countless individuals affected by DMD.

This case study showcases the immense potential of genetic engineering in the engineering field, particularly in the domains of biomedical science and biotechnology. It emphasizes the importance of interdisciplinary collaboration between engineers, scientists, and clinicians to address complex genetic disorders and develop innovative solutions.

By exploring this case study, engineers specializing in biomedical science and biotechnology can gain valuable insights into the engineering principles and techniques utilized in genetic engineering. It serves as an inspiration to push boundaries, think creatively, and leverage the power of precision engineering to tackle the most challenging problems in the field.

Ultimately, this case study reinforces the pivotal role of genetic engineering in the ongoing quest to improve human health and quality of life. As engineers, we have the opportunity to harness the potential of genetic engineering and gene therapy techniques to revolutionize the future of medicine and make a lasting impact on society.

Case Study 3: Gene Editing in Biomedical Engineering

Introduction:

In recent years, gene editing has emerged as a revolutionary tool in the field of biomedical engineering. This subchapter presents a fascinating case study on the applications, challenges, and potential of gene editing techniques in the realm of precision engineering. Engineers, particularly those specializing in biomedical science and biotechnology, will find this case study enlightening and inspiring as they explore the endless possibilities offered by gene editing in advancing healthcare and genetic therapies.

Case Study Overview:

This case study delves into the innovative applications of gene editing techniques and their impact on precision engineering in the biomedical field. We will examine the potential of gene editing in treating genetic diseases, developing targeted therapies, and improving the efficiency of gene delivery systems. Through this exploration, engineers will gain a comprehensive understanding of the intricate interplay between genetic engineering and biomedical science.

Applications of Gene Editing in Biomedical Engineering:

1. Treating Genetic Diseases: Gene editing offers a promising avenue for treating genetic disorders by modifying or correcting faulty genes. Engineers can leverage techniques like CRISPR-Cas9 to precisely edit the genome and rectify genetic mutations responsible for diseases such as cystic fibrosis, sickle cell anemia, and muscular dystrophy.

2. Targeted Therapies: With gene editing, engineers can develop customized treatment approaches for specific patients. By precisely editing genes involved in disease pathways, highly targeted therapies can be created, reducing side effects and improving patient outcomes.

3. Enhancing Gene Delivery Systems: One of the challenges in gene therapy is efficiently delivering therapeutic genes into target cells. Engineers can utilize gene editing techniques to optimize gene delivery systems, ensuring precise and effective delivery of therapeutic genes to the desired locations.

Challenges and Future Considerations:

While gene editing holds immense potential, it also presents ethical, societal, and technical challenges. Engineers must address concerns related to off-target effects, long-term safety, and equitable access to gene editing technologies. Furthermore, continued research and development are necessary to enhance the precision, efficiency, and affordability of gene editing techniques.

Conclusion:

Gene editing in biomedical engineering represents a groundbreaking frontier with immense potential to transform healthcare and genetic therapies. This case study has provided engineers specializing in biomedical science and biotechnology a comprehensive overview of the applications, challenges, and future considerations of gene editing techniques. By harnessing the power of precision engineering, engineers can contribute to the advancement of genetic engineering and gene therapy, ultimately improving the lives of countless individuals worldwide.

Chapter 11: Future Perspectives and Emerging Technologies in Genetic Engineering

Advancements in Gene Editing Techniques

In recent years, the field of gene editing has witnessed unprecedented breakthroughs, revolutionizing the way we approach genetic engineering and gene therapy. Engineers, particularly those specializing in biomedical science and biotechnology, play a crucial role in bringing these advancements to life. This subchapter aims to explore the most cutting-edge gene editing techniques and their potential applications in the realm of precision engineering.

One of the most significant advancements in gene editing is the development of CRISPR-Cas9 technology. CRISPR-Cas9, short for Clustered Regularly Interspaced Short Palindromic Repeats-CRISPR-associated protein 9, allows scientists to precisely modify specific genes within an organism's DNA. This technique acts as a molecular scissor, enabling engineers to edit DNA sequences with an unprecedented level of accuracy and efficiency. Its potential applications span across various domains, including medicine, agriculture, and biotechnology.

Another notable advancement is the emergence of base editing techniques. Traditionally, gene editing involved replacing specific DNA sequences, but base editing allows for precise alteration of individual nucleotides. By directly converting one base to another, this technique offers immense potential for correcting disease-causing mutations and enhancing desirable traits in various organisms. Engineers can harness this technology to design more effective gene therapies and create genetically modified organisms with enhanced productivity or resilience.

Furthermore, advancements in gene drive technology have opened up new possibilities for controlling and manipulating entire populations of organisms. Gene drives are genetic systems that can rapidly spread specific genes through a population, potentially altering entire ecosystems. Using gene editing techniques, engineers can introduce desired genetic modifications into target populations, such as disease-resistant mosquitoes or invasive plant species, effectively mitigating the impact of infectious diseases or invasive species on human health and the environment.

Lastly, the advent of prime editing presents yet another groundbreaking tool for precision gene editing. Prime editing combines the principles of CRISPR-Cas9 and reverse transcriptase to directly rewrite specific DNA sequences without requiring DNA breaks. This technique allows for precise insertions, deletions, or substitutions, expanding the possibilities for genetic modification. Engineers can leverage prime editing to correct disease-causing mutations in human cells or engineer specialized cells for therapeutic purposes.

As engineers continue to delve into these advancements, the potential for gene editing techniques to revolutionize healthcare, agriculture, and environmental conservation becomes increasingly evident. The ability to precisely modify genetic material offers unprecedented opportunities to tackle genetic diseases, enhance crop yields, and preserve biodiversity. However, it is crucial for engineers to approach these advancements with ethical considerations, ensuring responsible use and minimizing potential risks associated with unintended consequences.

In conclusion, the field of gene editing has witnessed remarkable advancements, providing engineers in the biomedical science and biotechnology niches with powerful tools for precision genetic engineering. With techniques like CRISPR-Cas9, base editing, gene drives, and prime editing, engineers can pave the way for groundbreaking applications in medicine, agriculture, and environmental conservation. By harnessing these advancements responsibly, engineers can contribute to a future where genetic diseases are eradicated, food security is enhanced, and ecosystems are preserved.

Synthetic Biology and Genetic Engineering

In recent years, the fields of biomedical science and biotechnology have witnessed remarkable advancements, thanks to the integration of precision engineering techniques with genetic engineering and synthetic biology. This subchapter aims to provide engineers with an in-depth understanding of these cutting-edge technologies and their applications in these two niches.

Synthetic biology can be defined as the engineering of biological systems or the design and construction of new biological parts, devices, and systems for useful purposes. Its emergence has revolutionized the way we think about genetic engineering by enabling scientists to engineer biological systems with unprecedented precision and control. By combining engineering principles with biology, synthetic biology offers a versatile toolkit for designing and constructing biological components, circuits, and even entire organisms.

Genetic engineering, on the other hand, involves the manipulation of an organism's genetic material to introduce desirable traits or modify existing ones. It encompasses a range of techniques, such as gene cloning, gene editing, and gene therapy, which play a crucial role in the fields of biomedical science and biotechnology. Genetic engineering techniques have been instrumental in developing new treatments for genetic disorders, creating genetically modified organisms (GMOs) for agricultural purposes, and producing recombinant proteins for therapeutic use.

Engineers in the fields of biomedical science and biotechnology can leverage these technologies to address a wide range of challenges. For instance, in the field of gene therapy, precision engineering techniques allow for the delivery of therapeutic genes into specific cells or tissues, offering potential cures for previously incurable diseases. Similarly, in biotechnology, synthetic biology empowers engineers to design and optimize microbial strains for the production of biofuels, pharmaceuticals, and industrial chemicals.

This subchapter will delve into the fundamental principles behind synthetic biology and genetic engineering, explaining the tools and methodologies employed in these fields. It will explore the ethical considerations associated with these technologies and highlight the potential risks and benefits. Moreover, it will showcase real-world applications and case studies that demonstrate the transformative power of precision engineering in biomedical science and biotechnology.

By equipping engineers with a comprehensive understanding of synthetic biology and genetic engineering, this subchapter aims to inspire innovation and encourage the integration of these technologies into their work. It serves as a guide for engineers, providing them with the knowledge and tools required to push the boundaries of biomedical science and biotechnology, ultimately leading to groundbreaking advancements that can improve human health and well-being.

Nanotechnology in Genetic Engineering

In recent years, the fields of biomedical science and biotechnology have witnessed remarkable advancements, thanks to the integration of nanotechnology into genetic engineering. The marriage of these two cutting-edge disciplines has opened up new possibilities and revolutionized the way we approach medical treatments and disease prevention. This subchapter aims to explore the impact of nanotechnology in genetic engineering, specifically addressing engineers in the fields of biomedical science and biotechnology.

Nanotechnology, the science of manipulating matter at the atomic and molecular scale, has provided engineers with powerful tools to manipulate and control genetic material. By harnessing nanoscale structures and devices, scientists can now precisely target and modify genes, paving the way for unprecedented breakthroughs in medicine.

One significant application of nanotechnology in genetic engineering is the targeted delivery of therapeutic agents. Nanoparticles, such as liposomes and polymeric nanoparticles, can be engineered to encapsulate and deliver genetic material directly to specific cells or tissues. This approach allows for precise gene editing, gene silencing, and gene replacement strategies, all of which hold immense potential for treating genetic disorders and combating diseases like cancer.

Moreover, nanotechnology has enabled the development of highly sensitive diagnostic tools. Nanosensors and nanodevices can detect and analyze genetic material in a rapid and accurate manner, leading to early disease detection and personalized medicine. These nanoscale sensors can detect specific DNA or RNA sequences, proteins, and other biomarkers, providing valuable information for disease diagnosis and monitoring.

Furthermore, nanotechnology has facilitated the creation of advanced gene delivery systems. Engineered nanocarriers can protect genetic material from degradation, enhance cellular uptake, and facilitate efficient gene transfer. These nanocarriers, such as viral vectors and nanoparticles, can be precisely tuned to optimize gene delivery, ensuring the desired therapeutic outcomes.

The integration of nanotechnology in genetic engineering has also revolutionized tissue engineering and regenerative medicine. Nanoscale materials and scaffolds can mimic the native tissue environment, providing a three-dimensional framework for cell growth and tissue regeneration. These nanomaterials can also release growth factors and other bioactive molecules to guide cellular behavior and promote tissue regeneration.

In conclusion, the combination of nanotechnology and genetic engineering has unleashed a new era of possibilities in the fields of biomedical science and biotechnology. Engineers now have the tools to precisely manipulate and control genetic material, leading to groundbreaking advancements in disease treatment, diagnosis, and tissue engineering. As nanotechnology continues to evolve, it is essential for engineers in these niches to stay abreast of the latest developments and embrace this powerful technology to drive innovation and improve human health.

Chapter 12: Conclusion and Final Thoughts

Recapitulation of Key Concepts

In this subchapter, we will recapitulate the key concepts discussed throughout the book "Precision Engineering: Exploring Genetic Engineering and Gene Therapy Techniques for Engineers." This book is specifically addressed to engineers, particularly those working in the niches of biomedical science and biotechnology. By revisiting the core concepts, we aim to reinforce your understanding and provide a comprehensive overview of the topics covered.

The book commenced with an introduction to genetic engineering, highlighting its significance in transforming the field of biotechnology. We discussed the fundamental principles of genetic engineering, including DNA structure, gene expression, and the central dogma of molecular biology. Understanding these concepts is crucial for engineers as they delve into genetic engineering techniques.

Next, we explored the various gene manipulation techniques used in genetic engineering. This included DNA cloning, polymerase chain reaction (PCR), and gene synthesis. We explained their underlying mechanisms, advantages, and limitations, empowering engineers to select the most appropriate technique for their research or application.

The subchapter on gene therapy techniques delved into the promising field of using genetic engineering to treat diseases. We explored the different approaches to gene therapy, such as gene addition, gene inhibition, and gene editing. Moreover, we discussed the challenges associated with gene therapy, including delivery methods and ethical considerations.

To ensure precision in genetic engineering, we dedicated a section to the emerging field of genome editing technologies. This included an in-depth explanation of CRISPR-Cas9, zinc finger nucleases (ZFNs), and transcription activator-like effector nucleases (TALENs). We highlighted their unique features, advantages, and potential applications.

Additionally, the book touched upon the importance of bioinformatics in genetic engineering. We emphasized the role of computational tools and databases in analyzing genetic data, designing experiments, and predicting gene functions. Understanding bioinformatics is crucial for engineers, as it enables them to leverage vast amounts of genetic information effectively.

Finally, we concluded the book by discussing the future prospects and challenges in precision engineering. We explored emerging trends, such as synthetic biology, personalized medicine, and gene drives. We also emphasized the importance of ethical considerations, safety protocols, and regulatory frameworks in the field of genetic engineering.

By recapitulating these key concepts, we aim to equip engineers in the biomedical science and biotechnology niches with a solid understanding of genetic engineering and gene therapy techniques. We hope that this knowledge will empower engineers to contribute to the advancement of precision engineering and drive innovation in the field.

Importance of Genetic Engineering and Gene Therapy for Engineers

Subchapter: Importance of Genetic Engineering and Gene Therapy for Engineers

Introduction:
In the rapidly advancing field of biomedical science and biotechnology, genetic engineering and gene therapy techniques have emerged as powerful tools for engineers. This subchapter aims to highlight the importance of these techniques and their relevance for engineers in these niches. By harnessing the potential of genetic engineering and gene therapy, engineers can contribute significantly to the development of innovative solutions to address complex medical challenges.

1. Accelerating Biomedical Research:
Genetic engineering allows engineers in the field of biomedical science and biotechnology to manipulate and modify genetic material with precision. By using techniques like CRISPR-Cas9, engineers can edit genes, enabling them to study diseases in greater detail and accelerating the discovery of potential therapies. This capability empowers engineers to make significant contributions to the field by providing valuable insights into disease mechanisms and facilitating the development of targeted treatments.

2. Designing Therapeutic Solutions:
Gene therapy, a cutting-edge approach, involves the modification or insertion of genes into a patient's cells to treat or prevent diseases. Engineers play a crucial role in designing and manufacturing the delivery systems for gene therapy, such as viral vectors or lipid

nanoparticles. Their expertise in precision engineering ensures the safe and effective delivery of therapeutic genes into the target cells, offering hope for patients suffering from genetic disorders, cancer, and other diseases.

3. Improving Diagnosis and Personalized Medicine: Genetic engineering techniques enable engineers to develop advanced diagnostic tools that can detect genetic variations associated with diseases. By designing and optimizing DNA sequencing technologies, engineers can contribute to the development of faster, more accurate, and cost-effective diagnostic methods. These advancements in diagnostics, combined with gene therapy, facilitate the emergence of personalized medicine, where treatments can be tailored to an individual's genetic makeup, leading to more effective and targeted therapies.

4. Overcoming Manufacturing Challenges: Engineers play a vital role in scaling up genetic engineering and gene therapy techniques for industrial production. By leveraging their expertise in process engineering, automation, and quality control, engineers can help overcome manufacturing challenges, ensuring consistent production of gene therapies and reducing costs. This contribution is essential to make these transformative therapies accessible to a larger population and maximize their impact.

Conclusion:
The importance of genetic engineering and gene therapy for engineers in the fields of biomedical science and biotechnology cannot be overstated. These techniques offer exciting opportunities to accelerate research, design therapeutic solutions, improve diagnostics, and

overcome manufacturing challenges. By embracing and leveraging these techniques, engineers can contribute significantly to the advancement of precision medicine, ultimately improving the lives of patients worldwide.

Future Potential and Challenges in the Field

In recent years, the field of precision engineering has witnessed remarkable advancements, particularly in the realm of genetic engineering and gene therapy techniques. These innovative approaches hold immense promise for engineers in the biomedical science and biotechnology sectors. With the potential to revolutionize healthcare and improve the quality of life for individuals with genetic disorders, the future looks incredibly bright. However, along with these opportunities come a host of challenges that engineers must confront to realize the full potential of this field.

One of the most significant potentials lies in the development of personalized medicine. Precision engineering techniques allow for the customization of treatments based on an individual's genetic makeup. By targeting specific genes responsible for diseases, engineers can design therapies that are tailored to a patient's unique genetic profile. This approach has the potential to enhance treatment efficacy while minimizing adverse effects, allowing for more efficient and personalized healthcare.

Moreover, precision engineering has the potential to eradicate hereditary diseases altogether. By utilizing gene therapy techniques, engineers can correct genetic mutations directly, offering hope for individuals suffering from inherited disorders. The ability to edit faulty genes or replace them with healthy copies could potentially eliminate diseases that have plagued humanity for generations.

Another area of immense potential lies in the field of regenerative medicine. Precision engineering techniques can be employed to manipulate stem cells, which have the remarkable ability to differentiate into various cell types. By directing their differentiation, engineers can generate tissues and organs that can be used for transplantation, addressing the shortage of organs available for patients in need. This advancement has the potential to revolutionize the field of organ transplantation and significantly improve patient outcomes.

However, along with these exciting prospects, precision engineering also faces several challenges. One major hurdle is the ethical considerations associated with gene editing. The ability to modify the human genome raises profound ethical questions regarding the limits and consequences of such interventions. Engineers must navigate these ethical dilemmas carefully to ensure that their work aligns with societal values and safeguards the well-being of individuals.

Additionally, the complexity of genetic systems and their interactions poses significant challenges. Engineers need to develop advanced computational models and algorithms to decipher the vast amount of genetic data and predict the outcomes of interventions accurately. The integration of engineering principles with biology and medicine is crucial for overcoming these challenges and advancing the field further.

In conclusion, precision engineering techniques in genetic engineering and gene therapy hold tremendous potential for engineers in the biomedical science and biotechnology sectors. The ability to personalize treatments, eradicate hereditary diseases, and advance regenerative medicine offers hope for a future with improved healthcare outcomes. However, engineers must navigate ethical considerations and overcome the complexities of genetic systems to fully realize the potential of this field. By rising to these challenges, engineers can shape a future where precision engineering techniques become integral to the advancement of healthcare and the betterment of society.

www.ingramcontent.com/pod-product-compliance
Lightning Source LLC
LaVergne TN
LVHW010555070526
838199LV00063BA/4981